DON'T MISS DR. D'ADAMO'S

Eat Right 4 Your Type
Complete Blood Type Encyclopedia:
The A–Z Reference Guide for the Blood Type
Connection to Symptoms, Disease, Conditions, Vitamins,
Supplements, Herbs and Food

NEARLY 1,000 ENTRIES ON TREATING SYMPTOMS
AND ILLNESS ACCORDING TO BLOOD TYPE

Learn how to treat everything from:

- Asthma to Thrombosis
- Allergies to Sore Throat

Discover how to treat over 300 conditions
using the *right remedy* for *your type*:

- Vitamins and Supplements
- Herbs and Food
- Exercise
- Stress Reduction
- Sleep and Regeneration

now available from Riverhead Books

BLOOD TYPE B

FOOD, BEVERAGE AND SUPPLEMENT LISTS

from

EAT RIGHT F4R YOUR TYPE

Dr. Peter J. D'Adamo
with Catherine Whitney

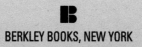

BERKLEY BOOKS, NEW YORK

THE BERKLEY PUBLISHING GROUP
Published by the Penguin Group
Penguin Group (USA) Inc.
375 Hudson Street, New York, New York 10014, USA
Penguin Group (Canada), 10 Alcorn Avenue, Toronto, Ontario M4V 3B2, Canada
(a division of Pearson Penguin Canada Inc.)
Penguin Books Ltd., 80 Strand, London WC2R 0RL, England
Penguin Group Ireland, 25 St. Stephen's Green, Dublin 2, Ireland (a division of Penguin Books Ltd.)
Penguin Group (Australia), 250 Camberwell Road, Camberwell, Victoria 3124, Australia
(a division of Pearson Australia Group Pty. Ltd.)
Penguin Books India Pvt. Ltd., 11 Community Centre, Panchsheel Park, New Delhi—110 017, India
Penguin Group (NZ), Cnr. Airborne and Rosedale Roads, Albany, Auckland 1310, New Zealand
(a division of Pearson New Zealand Ltd.)
Penguin Books (South Africa) (Pty.) Ltd., 24 Sturdee Avenue, Rosebank, Johannesburg 2196, South
Africa

Penguin Books Ltd., Registered Offices: 80 Strand, London WC2R 0RL, England

BLOOD TYPE B: FOOD, BEVERAGE AND SUPPLEMENT LISTS

A Berkley Book / published by arrangement with the authors

PRINTING HISTORY
Berkley edition / January 2002

Copyright © 2002 by Hoop-A-Joop, LLC.
Cover design by Steven Ferlauto.
Interior text design by Tiffany Estreicher.

ISBN: 0-425-18312-2

BERKLEY®
Berkley Books are published by The Berkley Publishing Group,
a division of Penguin Group (USA) Inc.,
375 Hudson Street, New York, New York 10014.
BERKLEY is a registered trademark of Penguin Group (USA) Inc.
The "B" design is a trademark belonging to Penguin Group (USA) Inc.

PRINTED IN THE UNITED STATES OF AMERICA

20 19 18 17 16 15 14 13 12 11

*To Blood Type Bs of the
Twenty-first Century, that you may fully realize
your remarkable heritage.*

Contents

Acknowledgments

There are many people to thank, as no scientific pursuit is solitary. Along the way, I have been driven, inspired, and supported by all of the people who placed their confidence in me. In particular, I give deep thanks to my wife, Martha, for her love and friendship; my daughters, Claudia and Emily, for the joy they bring me; and my parents, James D'Adamo Sr., N.D., and Christl, for teaching me to trust in my intuition.

I am also more grateful than I can express to:

Catherine Whitney, my writer, and her partner, Paul Krafin, who have transformed complex scientific ideas into accessible principles of everyday life;

My literary agent, Janis Vallely, whose commitment and wisdom are a continuing aid and inspiration;

Amy Hertz, my editor at Riverhead/Putnam, whose

vision and care have turned the blood type science into a meaningful mainstream program;

Jane Dystel, Catherine's literary agent, whose advice has been welcome;

Heidi Merritt, whose devotion and attention to detail have brought the manuscript closer to perfection;

My staff at 2009 Summer Street for their dedication and support, and the hardworking staff at 5 Brook Street;

All of the wonderful patients who in their quest for health and happiness chose to honor me with their trust.

What Type Bs Are Saying About the Diet

Michele W., 42

"I went on the Type B Diet on January 1, 1998, and I am still on it. I follow it strictly, and for the first three or four months I actually consumed more calories than I did before. I did this to test the diet. I knew if I cut my calories I would lose weight. I weighed 270 pounds and had half of my thyroid removed due to cancer over 20 years ago. I also had a problem with water retention. In the past, I had always handled water retention by consuming water, lemon juice, and cucumbers. But for about two months prior to my going on the diet, nothing that I tried worked. The Type B Diet reduced the water retention immediately by 80 percent. I have had great weight loss. As of today, I have lost 79 pounds and have 11 more to go."

Richard S., 53

"At the age of 53 I found it difficult to fight off the 'one pound a year syndrome' for people over 35. I exercised regularly and attempted to knock off the 10 pounds I'd gained. I have lost nine pounds in a month with few cravings. My mood has also lifted considerably. While I found the Atkins diet somewhat effective, it didn't give me enough stamina for my exercise routine. My wife was skeptical about this diet, but she is now quite supportive because of my mood change and weight loss."

Nancy R., 58

"I had been seeing a rheumatologist for extremely painful arthritis in my hips and knees. I also had difficulty in other joints, but these were the worst. After about 30 days on the Type B Diet, I began to notice significant pain relief. Now I have virtually no arthritis pain. Additionally, I have lost a significant amount of weight. I had lost weight before, however, and still had the arthritis. The exciting difference to me is the pain-free state I now enjoy!"

Ellen V., 33

"I suffered from chronic fatigue syndrome for several years, and it was ruining my life. My job performance was low, and I was in danger of losing my job. I couldn't exercise—something I had always enjoyed. I seemed to catch every bug that came along. I felt like an old woman! Every once in a while I

would start to feel better, and I'd be encouraged, but the malaise would always return. My naturopath recommended the Type B Diet, and I started it in May 1999. The improvement was immediate. I've been following the diet for a year now and I have my life back. I'm no longer fading out at work, I'm exercising, and best of all, my old optimism is back. Thank you, Dr. D'Adamo!"

Paul M., 45

"I had been struggling with what I felt was an immune deficiency, constantly battling recurring bouts of bronchitis, colds, flu, etc. Things finally reached a head when I was diagnosed with a hiatal hernia and was told that the only way to control it was through medication. I visited an acupuncturist who recommended that I try the Type B Diet. Before reading this book, I was eating chicken four to five times a week—roast chicken, chicken soup, chicken sandwiches . . . well, you get the idea. I thought it would be difficult to cut chicken out of my diet, but I started eating lamb in its place. While I didn't start this diet to lose weight, I lost about 10 pounds in two weeks, and this is without following the recommended portion size. The best thing, however, is that my overall health has improved. I no longer go through the day feeling like a slug, and people tell me that they can see the difference in my energy level. This is without even attempting to cut back on calories. While I was never really considered 'fat,' people tell me that they can see a big difference in my weight. The most amazing part is that

now my body feels that it can fight off common ailments. The last couple of times that I've started getting sick, I expected to wake up the next day feeling terrible. Amazingly, I would wake up and my symptoms would have all but disappeared. Even with the results that I've gotten, people are still skeptical. But who cares? I say. I feel great and I won't have to worry about my belly hanging out when we go to Hawaii."

A Message for Type Bs

Dear Type B Reader,

This special format book, Eat Right 4 Type B, *focuses on the principles and strategies of the Blood Type Diet as they apply to you. If you are new to the diet, you'll find this book to be a simple, accessible beginner's guide that will get you started on the basics. If you are already following the diet and have read the comprehensive series (*Eat Right 4 Your Type, Cook Right 4 Your Type, *and* Live Right 4 Your Type*), you'll find this book useful as a quick and portable reference guide for your diet.*

Since the introduction of the Blood Type Diet five years ago, I have received tens of thousands of testimonials from people all over the world. Many of them are from Type Bs who have overcome chronic health problems, serious illnesses, or lifelong struggles with weight

*merely by eating and living in accordance with the ge-
netic signals of their blood type. A growing body of research supports the conclusion that our individual
differences* do *matter when it comes to making strategic
health and lifestyle decisions.*

*I sincerely hope that you will join other Type Bs who
have had success with this plan. I invite you to share in
experiencing the renewed sense of well-being and good
health that have become reliable hallmarks of the Type
B Diet.*

Peter J. D'Adamo, N.D.

IMPORTANT NOTE

The contents of this book have been abridged to provide only the most basic information concerning the Blood Type Diet. To gain the full therapeutic benefit of the diet, it is important that you read Dr. D'Adamo's complete research and prescriptive advice as it appears in his three books, *Eat Right 4 Your Type, Cook Right 4 Your Type* and *Live Right 4 Your Type*. These books include extensive details that will help you fully understand the important role your blood type plays in determining diet, exercise, health, disease, longevity, physical vitality, and emotional stability.

The Blood Type–Diet Connection

The connection between blood type and diet is a new idea for most people, but they often find that it answers some of their most perplexing questions. We have long realized that there was a missing link in our comprehension of the process that leads either to the path of wellness or the path of disease. There had to be a reason why there were so many paradoxes in dietary studies and disease survival. Blood type analysis has given us a way to explain those paradoxes.

Blood types are as fundamental as creation itself. In the masterful logic of nature, the four blood types follow an unbroken trail from the earliest moment of human creation to the present day. They are the signatures of our ancient ancestors on the indestructible parchment of history. As Blood Type B, you carry the genetic imprint of your nomadic ancestors, who advanced the human race into uncharted territories. The Type B gene enabled your ancestors to survive and thrive at high elevations and in cold climates, with a balanced diet of meat, dairy, grains, and vegetables. Amazingly, at the beginning of the twenty-first century, your immune and digestive systems still maintain a predisposition for foods that your Type B ancestors ate.

Your blood type is the key to your body's entire immune system, and as such is the essential defining factor in your health profile. Your blood type antigen serves as the guardian at the gate, creating antibodies to ward off dangerous interlopers. When an antibody encounters the antigen of a microbial invader, a reaction called "agglutination" (literally, gluing) occurs. The antibody attaches to the viral antigen and makes it very sticky. When cells, viruses, parasites, and bacteria are agglutinated, they stick together and clump up, which makes the job of their disposal all the easier.

But there is much more to the agglutination story. Scientists have learned that many foods agglutinate the cells of certain blood types but not others, meaning that a food that may be harmful to the cells of one blood type may be beneficial to the cells of another.

A chemical reaction occurs between your blood and the foods that you eat. This reaction is part of your genetic inheritance. We know this because of a factor called "lectins." Lectins, abundant and diverse proteins found in foods, have agglutinating properties that affect your blood. Lectins are a powerful way for organisms in nature to attach themselves to other organisms in nature. Often, the lectins used by viruses or bacteria can be blood type specific, making them a stickier pest for a person of that blood type. Furthermore, when you eat a food containing protein lectins that are incompatible with your blood type antigen, the lectins target an organ or bodily system (kidneys, liver, brain, stomach, etc.) and begin to agglutinate blood cells in that area. For example, the lectin in chicken cross-reacts with Type B blood, targeting digestive enzymes and interfering with insulin production.

The Type B Diet is a way to restore the natural protective functions of your immune system, reset your metabolic clock, and clear your blood of dangerous agglutinating lectins. Depending on the severity of the condition, and the level of compliance with the plan, every person will realize some benefits from this diet.

THE TYPE B DIET BASICS

The key to the Type B Diet is balance. Type Bs thrive on the best that the animal and vegetable kingdoms have to offer. In a sense, Type B represents a sophisticated refinement in the evolutionary journey, an effort to join together divergent peoples and cultures. When you consume a balanced diet of meat, dairy, grains, and vegetables, you can control your weight and resist many of the most severe diseases common to modern life, such as heart disease and cancer.

The Type B Diet works because you are able to follow a clear, logical, scientifically researched and certified dietary blueprint based on your cellular profile.

Your diet is organized into fourteen food groups:

Meats and Poultry	**Vegetables**
Seafood	**Fruits**
Eggs and Dairy	**Juices and Fluids**
Oils and Fats	**Spices**
Nuts and Seeds	**Condiments**
Beans and Legumes	**Herbs and Herbal Teas**
Grains, Breads and Pasta	**Miscellaneous Beverages**

Within each group, food is divided into three categories: HIGHLY BENEFICIAL, NEUTRAL and AVOID. Think of the categories this way:

- **HIGHLY BENEFICIAL** is a food that acts like a **MEDICINE**.

• **AVOID** is a food that acts like a **POISON**.

• **NEUTRAL** is a food that acts like a **FOOD**.

The Type B Diet includes a wide variety of foods, so don't worry about limitations. When possible, show preference for the Highly Beneficial foods over the Neutral foods, but feel free to enjoy the Neutral foods that suit you; they won't harm you and they contain nutrients that are necessary for a balanced diet.

At the top of each food category, you will see a chart that looks something like this (note that the frequency is sometimes weekly, sometimes daily):

BLOOD TYPE B		Weekly, if your ancestry is . . .		
	PORTION	AFRICAN	CAUCASIAN	ASIAN
All seafood	4–6 oz.	1–4 x	3–5 x	4–6 x

The portion suggestions according to ancestry are not meant as firm rules. My purpose here is to present a way to fine-tune your diet even more, using what is known about the particulars of your ancestry. Although peoples of different races and cultures may share a blood type, they don't always have the same frequency of the gene. There are also geographic and cultural variations, as well as typical differences in the size and weight of various peoples. Use the refinements if you think they're helpful; ignore them if you find that they're not. In any case, try to formulate your own plan for portion sizes.

CHAPTER ONE

Meats and Poultry

BLOOD TYPE B		Weekly, if your ancestry is . . .		
	PORTION	AFRICAN	CAUCASIAN	ASIAN
Lean red meats	4–6 oz. (men)	3–4 x	2–3 x	2–3 x
Poultry	2–5 oz. (women and children)	0–2 x	0–3 x	0–2 x

There appears to be a direct connection between stress, autoimmune disorders, and red meat in the Type B system. That's because your Type B ancestors adapted better to other kinds of meats. (After all, there weren't a lot of steer on the Siberian tundra!) If you are fatigued or suffer from immune deficiencies, you should eat a red meat such as lamb, mutton, or rabbit several times a week, in preference to beef or turkey. In my experience, one of the most difficult adjustments Type Bs must make is to give up chicken. Chicken contains a Blood Type B agglutinating lectin in its muscle tissue. If you're accustomed to eating more poultry than red meat, you can eat other poultry such as turkey or pheasant.

HIGHLY BENEFICIAL

Goat	Rabbit
Lamb	Venison
Mutton	

NEUTRAL

Beef	Pheasant
Buffalo	Turkey
Liver	Veal
Ostrich	

AVOID

Bacon	Goose
Chicken	Grouse
Cornish hen	Guinea hen
Duck	Ham

AVOID (CONTINUED)

Heart	Quail
Horse	Squab
Partridge	Squirrel
Pork	Turtle

CHAPTER TWO

Seafood

BLOOD TYPE B		Weekly, if your ancestry is . . .		
	PORTION	AFRICAN	CAUCASIAN	ASIAN
All seafood	4–6 oz.	4–6 x	3–5 x	3–5 x

Type Bs thrive on seafood, especially the deep ocean fish like cod and salmon, which are rich in nutritious oils. White fish, such as flounder, halibut, and sole, are also excellent sources of high quality protein for Type Bs. Avoid all shellfish—crab, lobster, shrimp, mussels, etc. Shellfish contain lectins that are disruptive to the Type B system.

HIGHLY BENEFICIAL

Caviar (sturgeon)	Flounder
Cod	Grouper
Croaker	Haddock

HIGHLY BENEFICIAL (CONTINUED)

Hake	Pike
Halibut	Porgy
Harvest fish	Salmon
Mackerel	Sardine
Mahimahi	Shad
Monkfish	Sole
Ocean perch	Sturgeon
Pickerel	

NEUTRAL

Abalone	Drum
Bluefish	Grey sole
Bullhead	Herring (fresh)
Carp	Herring (kippers, pickled)
Catfish	Mullet
Chub	Muskellunge
Cusk	Opaleye fish

NEUTRAL (CONTINUED)

Orange roughy	Silver perch
Parrot fish	Smelt
Perch	Sole
Pompano	Squid (calamari)
Red snapper	Swordfish
Rosefish	Tilapia
Sailfish	Tilefish
Scallop	Tuna
Scrod	Weakfish
Scup	Whitefish
Shark	Whiting

AVOID

Anchovy	Butterfish
Barracuda	Clam
Bass (all types)	Conch
Beluga	Crab

AVOID (CONTINUED)

Crayfish	Oysters
Eel	Pollack
Frog	Shrimp
Lobster	Snail
Lox	Trout
Mussels	Turtle
Octopus	Yellowtail

CHAPTER THREE

Eggs and Dairy

BLOOD TYPE B		Weekly, if your ancestry is . . .		
	PORTION	AFRICAN	CAUCASIAN	ASIAN
Eggs	1 egg	3–4 x	3–4 x	5–6 x
Cheese	2 oz.	3–4 x	3–5 x	2–3 x
Yogurt	4–6 oz.	0–4 x	2–4 x	1–3 x
Milk	4–6 oz.	0–3 x	4–5 x	2–3 x

Type B is the only blood type that can fully enjoy a variety of dairy foods. That's because the primary sugar in the Type B antigen is D-galactosamine, the very same sugar present in milk. Dairy foods were first introduced to the human diet during the height of the Type B development, along with the domestication of animals. (By the way, eggs do not contain the lectin that is found in the muscle tissues of chicken.) However, there are ancestral idiosyncrasies that blur the picture. If you are of Asian descent, you may initially have a problem adapting to dairy foods—not because your system is resistant to them, but because your *culture* has typically been resistant. Dairy products were first introduced into Asian societies with the invasion of the Mongolian hordes. To the Asian mind, dairy products were the food of the barbarian, and thus not fit to eat. The stigma remains to this day, although there are large numbers of Type Bs in Asia whose soy-based diet is damaging to their systems. Type Bs of African descent might also have trouble adapting to dairy foods. Type Bs are barely represented in Africa, and many Africans are lactose intolerant.

HIGHLY BENEFICIAL

Cottage cheese	Milk (goat)
Farmer cheese	Mozzarella
Feta	Paneer
Goat cheese	Ricotta
Kefir	Yogurt
Milk (cow)	

NEUTRAL

Brie	Buttermilk
Butter	Camembert

NEUTRAL (CONTINUED)

Casein	Jarlsberg
Cheddar	Monterey jack
Colby	Muenster
Cream cheese	Neufchâtel
Edam	Parmesan
Egg (chicken)	Provolone
Emmenthal	Quark
Ghee (clarified butter)	Sherbet
Gouda	Sour cream
Gruyère	Swiss
Half & Half	Whey

AVOID

American cheese	Ice cream
Blue cheese	String cheese
Egg (duck, goose, quail)	

CHAPTER FOUR

Oils and Fats

BLOOD TYPE B		Weekly, if your ancestry is . . .		
	PORTION	AFRICAN	CAUCASIAN	ASIAN
Oils	1 tablespoon	3–5 x	4–6 x	5–7 x

Introduce olive oil into your diet to encourage proper digestion and healthy elimination. Use at least one tablespoon every other day. Avoid sesame, sunflower, and corn oils, which contain lectins that are damaging to the Type B digestive tract.

HIGHLY BENEFICIAL

Olive

NEUTRAL

Almond	Cod liver
Black currant seed	Evening primrose

NEUTRAL (CONTINUED)

Linseed (flaxseed)	Wheat germ
Walnut	

AVOID

Borage	Peanut
Canola	Safflower
Castor	Sesame
Coconut	Soy
Corn	Sunflower
Cottonseed	

CHAPTER FIVE

Nuts and Seeds

BLOOD TYPE B		Weekly, if your ancestry is . . .		
	PORTION	AFRICAN	CAUCASIAN	ASIAN
Nuts and seeds	Handful	2–3 x	2–3 x	2–3 x
Nut butters	1–2 tablespoons	2–4 x	2–4 x	2–4 x

Most nuts and seeds are not advised for Type Bs. Peanuts, sesame seeds, and sunflower seeds, among others, contain lectins that interfere with Type B insulin production. It might be difficult for Type B Asians to give up sesame seeds and sesame-based products, but in this case, your blood type speaks more definitively than your culture.

HIGHLY BENEFICIAL

Walnut (black)

NEUTRAL

Almond	Hickory
Almond butter	Linseed (flaxseed)
Beechnut	Lychee
Brazil	Macadamia
Butternut	Pecan
Chestnut	Walnut (English)

AVOID

Cashew	Poppy seed
Filbert	Pumpkin seed
Peanut	Sesame seed
Peanut butter	Sesame butter (tahini)
Pignola (pine)	Sunflower butter
Pistachio	Sunflower seed

CHAPTER SIX

Beans and Legumes

BLOOD TYPE B		Weekly, if your ancestry is . . .		
	PORTION	AFRICAN	CAUCASIAN	ASIAN
Beans and legumes	1 cup, dry	5–7 x	5–7 x	5–7 x

Type Bs can eat some beans and legumes, but many beans, such as lentils, garbanzos, pintos, and black-eyed peas, contain lectins that interfere with the production of insulin. Generally, Type B Asians tolerate beans and legumes better than other Type Bs because they are culturally accustomed to them.

HIGHLY BENEFICIAL

Kidney bean	Navy bean
Lima bean	

NEUTRAL

Broad bean	Northern bean
Cannellini bean	Red bean
Copper bean	Snap bean
Fava bean	String bean
Green bean	Tamarind bean
Green pea	White bean
Jícama bean	

AVOID

Adzuki bean	Soy cheese*
Black bean	Soy flakes*
Black-eyed pea	Soy granules*
Garbanzo bean (chickpea)	Soy milk*
Lentil	Soy, miso*
Mung bean/sprouts	Soy, tempeh*
Pinto bean	Soy, tofu*
Soy bean	

soy products

CHAPTER SEVEN

Grains, Breads and Pasta

BLOOD TYPE B		Weekly, if your ancestry is . . .		
	PORTION	AFRICAN	CAUCASIAN	ASIAN
Grains, breads and pasta	½ cup dry grains/ pasta, 1 muffin, 2 slices bread	5–7 x	5–9 x	5–9 x

I've encountered some Type Bs who can tolerate wheat products, but overall, they are like Type O in their intolerance. The wheat gluten contains a lectin that deposits in the muscle tissues, making them less efficient in burning calories and depressing the metabolic rate. Foods that are not quickly metabolized are stored as fat, so wheat can be a factor in Type B weight gain. Type Bs should also avoid rye, which contains a lectin that settles in your vascular system, causing blood disorders and, potentially, strokes. Corn and buckwheat are major factors in Type B weight gain. More than any other food, they contribute to a sluggish metabolism, insulin irregularity, fluid retention, and fatigue.

Try Essene or Ezekiel bread, found in health food stores. These "live" breads are highly nutritious. Although they contain sprouted wheat, the problem kernel is destroyed in the sprouting process, and they are quite digestible.

I would advise that you moderate your intake of breads, pasta and rice. You won't need much of these nutrients if you're consuming the meat, seafood and dairy products advised.

HIGHLY BENEFICIAL

Essene bread (manna bread)	Rice cake
Millet	Rice milk
Oat bran	Rice, puffed
Oatmeal	Spelt (whole)
Rice bran	

NEUTRAL

Barley	Ezekiel 4:9 Bread (100 percent sprouted)
Cream of Rice	Familia

NEUTRAL (CONTINUED)

Farina	Soy flour bread
Gluten-free bread	Spelt flour products
Granola	Spinach pasta
Grape-Nuts	Wheat (refined, unbleached)
Quinoa	Wheat (semolina flour products)
Rice bread	Wheat (white flour products)
Rice (white/brown/basmati)	Wheat bread, sprouted (not Essene/Ezekiel)
Rice flour	

AVOID

Amaranth	Corn (white/yellow/blue)
Artichoke pasta (pure)	Cornflakes
Barley	Cornmeal
Buckwheat/kasha	Couscous (cracked wheat)

AVOID (CONTINUED)

Cream of Wheat	Shredded wheat
Gluten flour	Soba noodles (100 percent buckwheat)
Grits	Sorghum
Kamut	Tapioca
Kasha popcorn	Teff
Rice (wild)	Wheat bran
Rye	Wheat germ
Rye bread (100 percent)	Wheat (gluten flour products)
Rye flour	Wheat (whole wheat products)
Seven grain bread/cereal	

CHAPTER EIGHT

Vegetables

BLOOD TYPE B		Daily, if your ancestry is . . .		
	PORTION	AFRICAN	CAUCASIAN	ASIAN
Cooked	1 cup, prepared	3–5 x	3–5 x	3–5 x
Raw	1 cup, prepared	3–5 x	3–5 x	3–5 x

There are many high-quality, nutritious vegetables available for Type Bs. Take full advantage of them with three to five servings a day. There is only a handful of vegetables that Type Bs should avoid, but take these guidelines to heart. Corn is filled with lectins that negatively affect your blood and digestion. Radishes and artichokes are also bad for Type B digestion. Tomatoes should be eliminated by Type Bs. Also avoid olives, since their molds can trigger allergic reactions. Since Type Bs tend to be more vulnerable to viruses and autoimmune diseases, eat plenty of leafy green vegetables, which contain magnesium, an important antiviral agent.

HIGHLY BENEFICIAL

Beets	Ginger
Beet greens	Kale
Broccoli	Mushroom, shiitake
Brussels sprouts	Mustard greens
Cabbage, all types	Parsley
Carrot	Parsnip
Cauliflower	Peppers, all types
Collard greens	Potato, sweet
Eggplant	Yam

NEUTRAL

Alfalfa sprouts	Broccoli rabe
Arugula	Caraway
Asparagus	Carrot juice
Asparagus pea	Celeriac
Bamboo shoots	Celery
Bok choy	Chervil

NEUTRAL (CONTINUED)

Chicory	Lettuce, all types
Chili pepper	Mushroom, abalone
Cilantro (coriander leaf)	Mushroom, enoki
Cucumber	Mushroom, maitake
Daikon radish	Mushroom, oyster
Dandelion	Mushroom, portobello
Dill	Mushroom, silver dollar
Endive	Okra
Escarole	Onion, all types
Fennel	Oyster plant
Fiddlehead fern	Pea (green, pod)
Garlic	Pickle (in brine or vinegar)
Horseradish	Pimiento
Kelp	Poi
Kohlrabi	Potato (all white-fleshed types)
Leek	Rappini

NEUTRAL (CONTINUED)

Rutabaga	String bean
Sauerkraut	Swiss chard
Scallion	Taro
Seaweed	Turnip
Shallot	Water chestnut
Snow pea	Watercress
Spinach	Yucca
Sprouts, alfalfa	Zucchini
Squash, all types (except pumpkin)	

AVOID

Artichoke, all types	Radish
Avocado	Rhubarb
Corn	Sprouts, mung bean
Olive, all types	Sprouts, radish
Pumpkin	Tomato

CHAPTER NINE

Fruits

BLOOD TYPE B		Daily, if your ancestry is . . .		
	PORTION	AFRICAN	CAUCASIAN	ASIAN
Recommended fruits	3–5 oz. or 1 fruit	3–4 x	3–4 x	3–4 x

There are very few fruits a Type B must avoid, and a wide range of beneficial fruits to choose from. Pineapple is especially good for Type Bs, who are susceptible to bloating—especially if you're not used to eating the dairy foods and meats on your diet. Bromelain, an enzyme in the pineapple, helps you to digest your food more easily. On the whole, you can choose your fruits liberally from the following lists.

Unless noted separately, all values of whole fruits apply to their juices as well.

HIGHLY BENEFICIAL

Banana	Pineapple
Cranberry	Plum, all types
Grape, all types	Watermelon
Papaya	

NEUTRAL

Apple/cider	Currant (black and red)
Apricot	Date
Asian pear	Dewberry
Blackberry	Elderberry
Blueberry	Fig (fresh/dried)
Boysenberry	Gooseberry
Breadfruit	Grapefruit
Canang melon	Guava
Cherry, all types	Honeydew melon
Christmas melon	Kiwi
Crenshaw melon	Kumquat

NEUTRAL (CONTINUED)

Lemon	Plantain
Lime	Prune
Loganberry	Quince
Mango	Raisin
Mulberry	Raspberry
Musk melon	Sago palm
Nectarine	Spanish melon
Orange	Strawberry
Peach	Tangerine
Pear	Youngberry
Persian melon	

AVOID

Bitter melon	Pomegranate
Coconut/milk	Prickly pear
Persimmon	Starfruit (carambola)

CHAPTER TEN

Juices and Fluids

BLOOD TYPE B		Daily, if your ancestry is . . .		
	PORTION	AFRICAN	CAUCASIAN	ASIAN
Recommended juices	8 oz.	2–3 x	2–3 x	2–3 x
Water	8 oz.	4–7 x	4–7 x	4–7 x

Most fruit and vegetable juices are okay for Type Bs. Choose vegetables and fruits according to the recommendations in chapters 8 and 9 when making or buying juice. In addition, I urge you to try the following beverage the first thing every morning as an immune and nervous system booster. I call it the "Membrane Fluidizer Cocktail," but I assure you that it's much more alluring than the name implies. Mix one tablespoon of flaxseed oil, one tablespoon of high-quality lecithin granules, and six to eight ounces of fruit juice. Shake and drink.

The Membrane Fluidizer Cocktail provides high levels of choline, serine, and ethanolamine (the phospho-

lipids), which are of great value to Type Bs. You may be
surprised to find that it's rather tasty, because the
lecithin emulsifies the oil, allowing it to mix with the
juice.

CHAPTER ELEVEN

Spices

Type Bs do best with warming herbs, such as ginger, horseradish, curry, and cayenne pepper. The exceptions are white and black pepper, which contain problem lectins. On the reverse side, sweet herbs tend to be stomach irritants, so avoid barley malt sweeteners, cornstarch, and cinnamon. The exceptions are white and brown sugar, honey, and molasses, which respond in a neutral way to the Type B digestive system. You may eat these sugars in moderation. You may also eat small quantities of chocolate, but try to consider it a condiment, not a main course!

HIGHLY BENEFICIAL

Cayenne pepper	Horseradish
Curry	Molasses (blackstrap)
Ginger	Parsley

NEUTRAL

Agar	Chervil
Anise	Chive
Apple pectin	Chocolate
Arrowroot	Clove
Basil	Coriander/leaf
Bay leaf	Cream of tartar
Bergamot	Cumin
Caper	Dill
Caraway	Dulse
Cardamom	Fructose
Carob	Garlic
Chili powder	Honey

NEUTRAL (CONTINUED)

Kelp	Sage
Mace	Sea salt
Maple syrup	Savory
Marjoram	Spearmint
Molasses	Sugar (white and brown)
Mustard (dry)	Tamari
Nutmeg	Tamarind
Oregano	Tarragon
Paprika	Thyme
Pepper, peppercorn	Turmeric
Pepper, red flakes	Vanilla
Peppermint	Vinegar, all types
Rice syrup	Wintergreen
Rosemary	Yeast (baker's/brewer's)
Saffron	

AVOID

Allspice	Gums (acacia, Arabic)
Almond extract	Juniper
Aspartame	Maltodextrin
Barley malt	Miso
Carrageenan	MSG
Cinnamon	Pepper, black and white
Cornstarch	Soy sauce
Corn syrup	Stevia
Gelatin, plain	Sucanat
Guarana	Tapioca

CHAPTER TWELVE

Condiments

Type Bs can handle just about every common condiment except ketchup (with its dangerous tomato lectins) and Worcestershire sauce (with its corn syrup), but common nutritional sense would suggest that you limit your intake of foods that provide no real benefit.

HIGHLY BENEFICIAL

None	

NEUTRAL

Jam (from acceptable fruits)	Jelly (from acceptable fruits)

NEUTRAL (CONTINUED)

Mayonnaise	Pickles, all types
Mustard	Salad dressing (from acceptable ingredients)
Pickle relish	

AVOID

Ketchup	Worcestershire sauce

CHAPTER THIRTEEN

Herbs and Herbal Teas

Ginseng is highly recommended for Type Bs because of its positive effect on the nervous system. Be aware, though, that it can act as a stimulant, so drink it early in the day. Licorice is particularly good for Type Bs. It has antiviral properties that work to reduce your susceptibility to autoimmune diseases. Also, many Type Bs experience a drop in blood sugar after meals (hypoglycemia), and licorice helps to regulate your blood sugar levels.

HIGHLY BENEFICIAL

Ginger	Peppermint
Ginseng	Raspberry leaf
Licorice	Rose hip
Parsley	Sage

NEUTRAL

Alfalfa	Mulberry
Burdock	Sarsaparilla
Catnip	Slippery elm
Cayenne	Spearmint
Chamomile	St. John's wort
Chickweed	Strawberry leaf
Dandelion	Thyme
Dong quai	Valerian
Echinacea	Vervain
Elder	White birch
Goldenseal	White oak bark
Hawthorn	Yarrow
Horehound	Yellow dock
Licorice root	

AVOID

Aloe	Cornsilk
Coltsfoot	Fenugreek

AVOID (CONTINUED)

Gentian	Rhubarb
Hops	Senna
Linden	Shepherd's purse
Mullein	Skullcap
Red clover	

CHAPTER FOURTEEN

Miscellaneous Beverages

Type Bs do best when you limit your beverages to herbal and green teas, water, and juice. Although beverages like coffee, regular tea, and wine do no real harm, the goal of the Type B Diet is to maximize your performance, not to keep it in neutral. If you're a caffeinated coffee or tea drinker, try replacing these beverages with green tea, which has caffeine but also provides some antioxidant benefits.

HIGHLY BENEFICIAL

Green tea

NEUTRAL

Beer	Tea, black regular/decaf
Coffee, regular or decaf	Wine, red/white

AVOID

Liquor	Seltzer water
Soda, all types	

CHAPTER FIFTEEN

Type B Supplement Advisory

Your Type B Plan also includes recommendations about vitamin, mineral and herbal supplements that can enhance the effects of your diet. As with food, nutritional supplements don't always work the same way for everyone. Every vitamin, mineral and herbal supplement plays a specific role in your body. The miracle remedy your Type A friend raves about may be inert or even harmful for your Type B system.

Your goal for any kind of supplementation is to enhance your Type B strengths and add an additional barrier of protection against your weaknesses. Therefore, your targeted focus should be:

- Fine-tuning an already balanced diet.

- Improving insulin production.

- Strengthening viral immunity.

- Improving brain clarity and focus.

The following recommendations emphasize the supplements that help to meet these goals. There are no supplements that are of particular harm to Type Bs. The key is balance. For the most part, you can avoid major diseases by following your Type B Diet. Because your diet is so rich in vitamin A, vitamin B, vitamin E, vitamin C, calcium, and iron, there is little need for supplementation of these vitamins and minerals.

BENEFICIAL

Magnesium

For Type Bs, there is a special risk of magnesium deficiency. That's because you are so efficient in assimilating calcium that you risk creating an imbalance between your levels of calcium and magnesium. Should this occur, you find yourself more at risk for viruses (or otherwise lowered immunity), fatigue, depression, and potentially, nervous disorders. In these instances, perhaps a trial of magnesium supplementation (300–500 mg) should be considered. Also, many Type B children are plagued with eczema, and magnesium

supplementation can often be beneficial. Any form of
magnesium is fine, although more patients report a lax-
ative effect with magnesium citrate than with the other
forms.

BEST MAGNESIUM-RICH FOODS FOR TYPE BS:

**all recommended green vegetables, grains,
and legumes**

HERBS/PHYTOCHEMICALS

Licorice (*Glycyrrhiza glabra*). Licorice is a plant
widely used by herbalists around the world. It contains
at least four benefits—as a treatment for stomach ulcers,
as an antiviral agent against the herpes virus, to treat
chronic fatigue syndrome, and to combat hypoglycemia. Licorice is a plant to be respected: large doses
can cause sodium retention and elevated blood pressure.
If you suffer from hypoglycemia, a condition in which
the blood sugar drops after a meal, drink a cup or two of
licorice tea after meals. If you suffer from chronic fatigue syndrome, I recommend that you use licorice
preparations, other than DGL and licorice tea, only un-
der the guidance of a physician. Licorice freely used in
its supplemental form can be toxic.

Digestive enzymes. If you are not used to eating meat or dairy foods, you may experience some initial difficulties adapting to your diet. Take a digestive enzyme with your main meals for a while, and you'll adjust more readily to concentrated proteins. Bromelain, an enzyme found in pineapples, is available in supplemental form at many health-food stores, usually in the 4X strength.

Adaptogenic herbs. Adaptogenic herbs increase concentration and memory retention, sometimes a problem for Type Bs with nervous or viral disorders. The best are Siberian ginseng (*Eleutherococcus senticosus*) and gingko biloba, both widely available in pharmacies and health-food stores. Siberian ginseng has been shown in Russian studies to increase the speed and accuracy of Teletype operators. Gingko biloba increases the microcirculation to the brain, which is why it is often prescribed to the elderly. It is currently being promoted as a brain stimulant, a pick-me-up for the mind.

Lecithin. Lecithin, a blood enhancer found principally in soy, allows the cell surface B antigens to move around more easily and better protect the immune system. Type Bs should seek this benefit from lecithin granules, not soy itself, as soy doesn't have the concentrated effect. Take the Membrane Fluidizer Cocktail, recommended in the Type B Diet.

CHAPTER SIXTEEN

Medical Strategies

Modern science has presented the medical community with a bewildering array of medications, and all of them are being prescribed by well-meaning physicians world-wide. But have we been careful enough in our use of antibiotics and vaccines? How do you know which medications are best for you, for your family, for your children? Again, blood type holds the answer.

As a naturopathic physician, I try to avoid prescribing over-the-counter medications. In most cases, there are natural alternatives that work just as well or better—and they don't have some of the problematic side effects of many pharmaceutical preparations.

The following natural remedies are safe for Type B:

ARTHRITIS

alfalfa

boswella

calcium

epsom salt bath

rosemary tea soak

CONGESTION

licorice tea

nettle

vervain

CONSTIPATION

fiber

larch tree bark (ARA-6)

psyllium

slippery elm

COUGH

horehound

CRAMPS, GAS

chamomile tea

fennel tea

ginger

peppermint tea

probiotic supplement with bifidus factor

DIARRHEA

blueberries

elderberries

L. acidophilus (yogurt culture)

raspberry leaf

EARACHE

garlic-mullein-olive-oil eardrops

FEVER

catnip

feverfew

vervain

white willow bark

FLU

garlic

arabinogalactan

rose hip tea

HEADACHE

chamomile

damiana

feverfew

valerian

white willow bark

INDIGESTION, HEARTBURN

bromelain

gentian

ginger

peppermint

MENSTRUAL CRAMPS

Jamaican dogwood

NAUSEA

ginger

licorice root tea

cayenne

SINUSITIS

thyme

SORE THROAT

stone root

TOOTHACHE

crushed-garlic gum massage

oil-of-cloves gum massage

CHAPTER SEVENTEEN

Frequently Asked Questions

Do I have to make all of the changes at once for my Type B Diet to work?

No. On the contrary, I suggest you start slowly, gradually eliminating the foods that are not good for you and increasing those that are highly beneficial. Many diet programs urge you to plunge in headfirst and radically change your life immediately. I think it's more realistic and ultimately more effective if you engage in a learning process. Don't just take my word for it. You have to "learn" it in your body. Before you begin your Type B Diet, you may know very little about which foods are good or bad for you. You're used to making your choices according to your taste buds, family traditions, and fad diet books. Chances are you are eating some foods that are good for you, but the Type B Diet provides you with a powerful tool for making informed choices every time. Once you know what your optimal eating plan is, you have the freedom to veer from your diet on occasion. Rigidity is the enemy of joy; I certainly am not a proponent of it. The Type B Diet is designed to make you feel great, not miserable and deprived. Obviously, there are going to be times when common sense tells you to relax the rules a bit—such as when you're eating at a relative's house.

Why do you list different portion recommendations according to ancestry?

The portions listings according to ancestry are merely refinements to the diet that you may find helpful. In the same way that men, women, and children have different portion standards, so, too, do people according to their body size and weight, geography, and cultural food preferences. These suggestions will help you get started until you are comfortable enough with the diet to naturally eat the appropriate portions. The portion recommendations also take into account specific problems that people of different ancestries tend to have with food. African Americans, for example, are often lactose intolerant, and most Asians are not accustomed to eating dairy foods, so they may have to introduce these foods slowly to avoid negative reactions.

Must I eat all of the foods marked "highly beneficial"?

It would be impossible to eat everything on your diet! Think of your Blood Type Diet as a painter's palette from which you may choose colors in different shades and combinations. However, do try to reach the weekly amount of the various food groups, if possible. Frequency is probably more important than the individual portions. If you have a small build, reduce the size of your portions, but maintain a regular frequency. This will ensure that the most valuable nutrients will continue to be delivered into the blood stream at a constant rate.

What should I do if an "avoid" food is the fourth or fifth ingredient in a recipe?

That depends on the severity of your condition, or the degree of your compliance. If you have food allergies, or colitis, you may want to practice complete avoidance. Many high-compliance patients avoid these foods altogether, although I think this might be too extreme. Unless you suffer from a specific allergic condition, it won't hurt most people to occasionally eat a food that is not on their diet.

Will I lose weight on the Blood Type Diet?

There are several ways to answer that question. First, most people who are overweight are eating an imbalanced diet—foods that upset metabolism, hamper proper digestion, and cause water retention. These are all factors that lead to overweight. The Blood Type Diet is the ultimate *balanced* diet, specifically tailored for you. If you follow your Blood Type Diet, your metabolism will adjust to its normal level and you'll burn calories more efficiently; your digestive system will process nutrients properly and reduce water retention. In time, perhaps a very short time, your weight will adjust accordingly. In my practice, I've found that most of my patients who have weight problems also have a history of chronic dieting. One would think that constant dieting would lead to weight loss, but that's not true if the structure of the diet and the foods it includes go against everything that makes sense for your specific body type. In our culture, we tend to promote "one size fits all" weight-loss programs, and then we wonder why they don't work. The answer is obvious! Different blood types respond to food in different ways. For example, Type Bs are able to metabolize many dairy foods healthfully, while the same foods lead to digestive and immune problems in Type Os and Type As. If you want to lose weight, your Blood Type Diet will tell you how.

Do calories matter on the Blood Type Diet?

There is an adjustment period on this diet, and over time you'll be able to adjust food amounts according to your needs. It's important to be aware of portion sizes. No matter *what* you eat, if you eat *too much* of it you'll gain weight. This probably seems so obvious that it doesn't even bear mentioning. But overeating has become one of America's most difficult and dangerous health problems. Millions of Americans are bloated and dyspeptic because of the amounts of food they eat. When you eat excessively, the walls of your stomach stretch like an inflated balloon. Although stomach muscles are elastic and were created to contract and expand, when they are grossly enlarged the cells of the abdominal walls undergo a tremendous strain. If you are eating until you feel full, and you normally feel sluggish after a meal, try to reduce your portion sizes. Learn to listen to what your body is telling you.

I've never heard of many of the grains you mention. Where do I find out more?

If you're looking for alternative grains, health-food stores are a bonanza. In recent years, many ancient grains, largely forgotten, have been rediscovered and are now being produced. Examples of these are amaranth, a grain from Mexico, and spelt, a variation of wheat that seems to be free of the problems found with whole wheat. Try them! They're not bad. Spelt flour makes a hearty, chewy bread that is quite flavorful, while several interesting breakfast cereals are now being made with amaranth. Another alternative is to use sprouted wheat breads, sometimes referred to as "Ezekiel" or "Essene" bread, as the gluten lectins found principally in the seed coat are destroyed by the sprouting process. These breads spoil rapidly and are usually found in the refrigerator cases of health-food stores. They are a "live" food, with many beneficial enzymes still intact. (Beware of comercially produced "sprouted wheat" breads, as they usually have a minority of sprouted wheat and a majority of whole wheat in their formulas.) Sprouted wheat breads are somewhat sweet tasting, as the sprouting process also releases sugars, and are moist and chewy. They make wonderful toast.

Is there an exercise recommendation for Type Bs?

Type Bs do well with exercises that are neither too aerobically intense nor completely aimed at mental relaxation. The ideal balance is a program composed of moderate activities that involve other people, such as group hiking, biking excursions, the less aggressive martial arts, tennis, and aerobics classes. You don't do as well when the sport is fiercely competitive—such as squash, football, or basketball. The most effective exercise schedule for Type Bs would be three days a week of more intense physical activity, and two days a week of relaxation exercises, such as yoga.

Type B at a Glance

TYPE B
The Nomad
balanced · flexible · creative

STRENGTHS	WEAKNESSES	MEDICAL RISKS
Strong immune system	No natural weaknesses. However, imbalance causes tendency toward autoimmune disease and rare, slow-growing viruses	Type I diabetes
Versatile adaptation to dietary and environmental changes		Chronic fatigue syndrome
Balanced nervous system		Autoimmune diseases: Lou Gehrig's disease, lupus, multiple sclerosis

DIET PROFILE	WEIGHT LOSS KEY	SUPPLEMENTS	EXERCISE REGIMEN
BALANCED OMNIVORE	AVOID	Magnesium	Moderate
	Chicken	Licorice	physical
	Corn	Ginkgo	exercise,
Meat	Lentil	biloba	with a
Dairy	Peanuts	Lecithin	mental
Grains	Sesame		component,
Vegetables	seeds		such as
Fruit	Buckwheat		hiking,
	Wheat		cycling,
			tennis, and
	USE		swimming
	Greens		
	Eggs		
	Venison		
	Liver		
	Licorice		
	tea		

Blood Type Learning Center

Now that you're familiar with the basic principles of the Blood Type Diet, I encourage you to expand your level of learning and application. The "right for your type" series offers the most comprehensive, scientifically grounded, and clinically tested information available on the four blood types. In order to truly make the most of your individualized diet and lifestyle recommendations, it's important for you to have a working knowledge of all four blood types. Your differences do not exist in a vacuum, but are part of nature's complex system of opposition and synergism. Your understanding of the evolutionary factors that distinguish the blood types will enhance your ability to live more fully as a Type B. In addition, these books offer extensive additional information and recommendations about your blood type. The series includes:

Live Right 4 Your Type
The Individualized Prescription for
Maximizing Health, Metabolism, and
Vitality in Every Stage of Your Life
by Dr. Peter J. D'Adamo, with Catherine Whitney
(G. P. Putnam's Sons, 2001)
Also available on audiocassette

In *Live Right 4 Your Type*, Dr. D'Adamo shows how living according to blood type can help people achieve total physical and emotional health at every stage of life. Aided by cutting-edge genetic research and the documentation of hundreds of research studies, Dr. D'Adamo presents readers with a life-enhancing program, which includes:

· The latest discoveries about the genetics of blood type and how they affect the body's systems.
· A study of the role of subtypes, in particular secretor status.
· Groundbreaking data on the connection between blood type and stress, personality, and mental health.
· A thorough investigation of the variations in digestion, metabolism, and immunity, depending on blood type.
· Individualized blood type prescriptions that show how to make lifestyle adaptations, reduce stress,

gain emotional balance, slow down aging, and avoid disease.
- Targeted advice for children, seniors, and women.
- Extensive research notes, patient outcomes, and resources.

Eat Right 4 Your Type
The Individualized Diet Solution to
Staying Healthy, Living Longer &
Achieving Your Ideal Weight
by Dr. Peter J. D'Adamo, with Catherine Whitney
(G. P. Putnam's Sons, 1996)
Also available on audiocassette

Eat Right 4 Your Type is Dr. D'Adamo's ground-breaking book, which first introduced the concept of the connection between blood type, diet, and health to a mass audience. With over two million copies in print and translated into fifty languages, *Eat Right 4 Your Type* remains the seminal work in the field. It includes:

- A detailed exploration of the anthropological and biological origins of the blood types.
- Comprehensive diet, exercise and meal plans for each blood type.
- Special recommendations for medical problems, weight loss, aging, infertility, and other issues.

- Case histories from Dr. D'Adamo's clinic, showing the remarkable results of the Blood Type Diet.
- An extensive bibliography, research and support section.

Cook Right 4 Your Type
The Practical Kitchen Companion to
Eat Right 4 Your Type
by Dr. Peter J. D'Adamo, with Catherine Whitney
(G. P. Putnam's Sons, 1998)

Cook Right 4 Your Type is the essential guide for living with and enjoying your Blood Type Diet. With the assistance of a team of professional chefs, Dr. D'Adamo presents a book chock-full of vital information and delicious recipes for each blood type. The book features:

- Food lists and shopping guides to help you set up your kitchen.
- Family-friendly recipe charts that show how to cook for more than one blood type.
- Hundreds of tips and practical guidelines for eating right for your type.
- 30-day meal plans to help integrate the diet into daily life.
- More than 200 original recipes to please every blood type palate.

Resources and Support

DR. PETER J. D'ADAMO: PATIENT SERVICES

Dr. Peter D'Adamo and his staff continue to accept new patients on a limited basis. To find out more about scheduling an appointment, please contact:

The D'Adamo Clinic
2009 Summer Street
Stamford, CT 06905
203-348-4800

Note: Please do not submit questions regarding Dr. D'Adamo's work or seeking personal advice on health matters.

ON THE WEB: WWW.DADAMO.COM

The World Wide Web has proven to be a valuable venue for exploring and applying the tenets of the Blood Type Diet and lifestyle. Since January 1997 hundreds of thousands have visited the site to participate in the ABO chat groups, to peruse the scientific archives, to share experiences and recipes, and to learn more about the science of blood type. The Web site has an interactive message board and archives of past posts to the board.

One of the most important features on the Web page is the Blood Type Outcome Registry, which has facilitated the collection of data on the measurable effects of the Blood Type Diet on a wide range of medical conditions. Visitors are encouraged to share their results.

SELF-TESTING SERVICES

North American Pharmacal, Inc., is the official distributor of Home Blood Type Testing Kits. Each kit costs $7.95 and is a single-use disposable educational device capable of determining one individual's ABO and rhesus blood type. Results are obtained within four to five minutes. If you have several friends or family members who need to learn their blood type, you will need to order a separate home blood-typing kit for each individual.

All U.S. orders are shipped via UPS ground (shipping

and handling cost is $5.25 per order irrespective of the number of kits ordered). Expedited shipping methods (UPS second day or next day) are available but cost more. Please contact the customer service department to inquire about rates for expedited shipping to your area.

If you are ordering a kit to be shipped outside of the U.S., shipping rates can vary dramatically and can be quite expensive. Please contact our customer service department prior to placing your order for an estimate of shipping charges for non-U.S. orders.

To order a single Home Blood Typing Kit please enclose $7.95 + $5.25 for shipping and handling and send to:

North American Pharmacal, Inc.
5 Brook Street
Norwalk, CT 06851
Tel: 203-866-7664
Fax: 203-838-4066
Toll free: 877-ABO TYPE (877-226-8973)
www.4yourtype.com

North American Pharmacal, Inc., offers a range of other self-tests to monitor aspects of health such as stress hormone levels, female hormone levels, mineral balance, and antioxidant status. There is also a test to determine secretor status. For prices and ordering information please contact North American Pharmacal.

BLOOD TYPE PRODUCTS AND SUPPLEMENTS

North American Pharmacal, Inc., is the official distributor of Blood Type Specialty Products. The product line includes supplements, books, tapes, teas, meal replacement bars, cosmetics, and support material that makes eating and living right for your type easier. Included in this product line are: New Chapter® D'Adamo 4 Your Type Products™. These whole-food vitamins, herbs, and other food supplements have been specifically crafted to address the unique requirements of each blood type.

Also included are Sip Right 4 Your Type™ teas, Deflect™ lectin-blocking formulas, and a range of additional blood-type-specific and blood-type-friendly health products that have been formulated in partnership with The Republic of Tea and New Chapter.

Product information and price lists are available from:

North American Pharmacal, Inc.
5 Brook Street
Norwalk, CT 06851
Tel: 203-866-7664
Fax: 203-838-4066
Toll free: 877-ABO-TYPE (877-226-8973)
www.4yourtype.com